THE BRAIN HEALTH DIET RECIPES COOKBOOK

GEORGE ANDERSON

CHAPTER ONE

INTRODUCTION

Brain

A brain is an organ that serves as the center of the nervous system in all vertebrate and most invertebrate animals. It is located in the head, usually close to the sensory organs for senses such as vision. It is the most complex organ in a vertebrate's body. In a human, the cerebral cortex contains approximately 14–16 billion neurons, and the estimated number of neurons in the cerebellum is 55–70 billion. Each neuron is connected by synapses to several thousand other neurons. These neurons typically communicate with one another by means of long fibers called axons, which carry trains of signal pulses called action potentials to distant parts of the brain or body targeting specific recipient cells.

Physiologically, brains exert centralized control over a body's other organs. They act on the rest of the body both by generating patterns of muscle activity and by driving the secretion of chemicals called hormones. This centralized control allows rapid and coordinated responses to changes in the environment. Some basic types of responsiveness such as reflexes can be mediated by the spinal cord or peripheral ganglia, but sophisticated purposeful control of behavior based on complex sensory input requires the information integrating capabilities of a centralized brain.

The operations of individual brain cells are now understood in considerable detail but the way they cooperate in ensembles of millions is yet to be solved. Recent models in modern neuroscience treat the brain as a biological computer, very different in mechanism from an electronic computer, but similar in the sense that it acquires information from the surrounding world, stores it, and processes it in a variety of ways.

This article compares the properties of brains across the entire range of animal species, with the greatest attention to vertebrates. It deals with the human brain insofar as it shares the properties of other brains. The ways in which the human brain differs from other brains are covered in the human brain article. Several topics that might be covered here are instead covered there because much more can be said about them in a human context. The most important that are covered in the human brain article are brain disease and the effects of brain damage.

Anatomy and function

Cerebrum

The cerebrum is the largest part of the brain. It's divided into two halves, called hemispheres.

The two hemispheres are separated by a groove called the great longitudinal fissure. The corpus callosum connects the two hemispheres, thus allowing the brain to deliver messages from one side to the other.

Each hemisphere of the cerebrum is divided into broad regions called lobes. Each lobe is associated with different functions:

• Frontal lobes. The frontal lobes are the largest of the lobes. As indicated by their name, they're located in the front part of the brain. They coordinate high-level behaviors, such as motor skills, problem-solving, judgment, planning, and attention. The frontal lobes also manage emotions, personality, and temper.

• Parietal lobes. The parietal lobes are located behind the frontal lobes. They're involved in organizing and interpreting sensory information from other parts of the brain.

• Temporal lobes. The temporal lobes house the auditory cortex. They are located on either side of the head on the same level as the ears. They coordinate specific functions, including hearing, visual memory (such as facial recognition), verbal memory (such as understanding language), and interpreting the emotions and reactions of others.

• Occipital lobes. The occipital lobes are located in the back of the brain. They're heavily involved in the ability to read and recognize colors and shapes.

Cerebellum

The cerebellum is located in the back of the brain, just below the occipital lobes. It's involved with fine motor skills, which refers to the coordination of smaller, or finer, movements, especially those involving the hands and feet.

The cerebellum also helps the body maintain its posture, equilibrium, and balance.

Diencephalon

The diencephalon is located at the base of the brain. It contains the:

• thalamus

• subthalamus

• epithalamus

• hypothalamus

The thalamus acts as a kind of relay station for signals coming into the brain. It's also involved in alertness, pain sensations, and attention.

The epithalamus serves as a connection between the limbic system and other parts of the brain. The limbic system is a part of the brain that's involved with emotion.

The hypothalamus processes information that comes from the autonomic nervous system. Its role includes controlling eating, sleeping, and sexual behavior. Some specific actions the hypothalamus is responsible for include:

• maintaining daily physiological cycles, such as the sleep-wake cycle

• controlling appetite

• regulating body temperature

• controlling the production and release of hormones

Brain stem

The brain stem is located in front of the cerebellum and connects to the spinal cord. It's responsible for passing messages to various parts of the body and the cerebral cortex. It consists of three major parts:

• Midbrain. The midbrain helps control eye movement, processes visual and auditory information, regulates motor movements, and is involved in arousal and wakefulness.

• Pons. This is the largest part of the brain stem. It's located below the midbrain. It's a group of nerves that help connect different parts of the brain. The pons also contains the start of some of the cranial nerves. These nerves are involved in facial movements and transmitting sensory information, as well as breathing.

• Medulla oblongata. The medulla oblongata is the lowest part of the brain. It acts as the connection between the brain stem and spinal cord. It also acts as the control center for the function of the heart and lungs. It helps regulate many important functions, including motor and sensory functions, breathing, sneezing, and swallowing.

Brain conditions

There are hundreds of conditions that can affect the brain. Most of them fall within 1 of 5 main categories:

• brain injuries, such as concussions

• cerebrovascular injuries, such as aneurysms or strokes

• brain tumors, such as acoustic neuromas or schwannomas

• neurodegenerative disorders, such as dementia, Parkinson's disease, or Huntington's disease

• psychological conditions, such as anxiety, depression, or schizophrenia

Symptoms of a brain condition

The brain is one of your most important body parts, so it's important to know how to recognize signs that there may be a problem.

Brain injury symptoms

Brain injury symptoms depend on the type and severity of the injury. While they sometimes appear immediately after a traumatic event, they can also show up hours or days later.

General brain injury symptoms may include:

• headache

• nausea or vomiting

• feeling confused or disoriented

• dizziness

• feeling tired or drowsy

• speech problems, including slurring

• sleeping more or less than usual

• dilation of one or both pupils

• inappropriate emotional responses

• seizures

• sensory problems, such as blurry vision or a ringing in your ears

• trouble remembering things or difficulty concentrating

• extreme mood changes or unusual behavior

Cerebrovascular injury symptoms

Symptoms tend to come on suddenly and include:

• severe headache

• loss of vision

• inability to speak

• inability to move or feel a part of the body

• drooping face

• coma

Brain tumor symptoms

Brain tumor symptoms depend on the size, location, and type of tumor.

General brain tumor symptoms may include:

• headache

• nausea or vomiting

• loss of motor coordination, such as trouble walking

- feeling sleepy

- feelings of weakness

- appetite changes

- convulsions or seizures

- issues with your vision, hearing, or speech

- difficulty concentrating

- extreme mood changes or behavior changes

Neurodegenerative symptoms

Neurodegenerative diseases cause damage to nervous tissue over time, so their symptoms may get worse as time goes on.

General neurodegenerative symptoms include:

- memory loss or forgetfulness

- changes in mood, personality, or behavior

- issues with motor coordination, such as difficulty walking or staying balanced

• speech issues, such as slurring or hesitation before speaking

Psychological symptoms

Symptoms of psychological, or mental health, conditions can be very different from person to person, even when they involve the same condition.

Some general symptoms of a mental health condition include:

• excessive feelings of fear, worry, or guilt

• feeling sad or dejected

• confusion

• difficulty concentrating

• low energy

• extreme stress that gets in the way of daily activities

• extreme mood changes

• withdrawal from loved ones or activities

• delusions or hallucinations

- suicidal ideation

Tips for a healthy brain

Some brain conditions may be outside your control, like trauma to the brain or mental health issues.

But there are things you can control and do to help keep your brain in good health, and to reduce your risk of certain health conditions.

Protect your head

Always wear a helmet when playing contact sports or riding a bike. Be sure to buckle up when you get in the car. Both of these can go a long way when it comes to avoiding brain injuries.

Exercise

Doing regular cardio workouts stimulates blood flow throughout your body, including your brain. It can also improve brain health in a variety of ways, including:

- improved emotional health

- improved learning ability

• reduced anxiety

• reduced cognitive decline

Quit smoking

Smoking isn't great for your overall health. That includes your brain: Smoking may lead to cognitive decline.

Listen to your thoughts

Try to check in from time to time with your thoughts or feelings. Keeping a diary is a good way to get into this habit. Look for any thought patterns or emotions that seem to be impacting your day-to-day life. They could be a sign of an underlying, treatable mental health condition.

Focus on a nutritious diet

What you eat can have a direct impact on the health of your brain, especially as you age. Many of the foods that are often recommended for brain health include lots of greens, fruits, nuts, fish, whole grains, olive oil and, occasionally, wine.

CHAPTER TWO

DEFINITION OF BRAIN HEALTH

Currently, there is no universally recognised definition of brain health. Most existing definitions have only a general description of normal brain function or emphasise one or two dimensions of brain health. The US Centers for Disease Control and Prevention defined brain health as an ability to perform all the mental processes of cognition, including the ability to learn and judge, use language, and remember. The American Heart Association/American Stroke Association (AHA/ASA) presidential advisory defined optimal brain health as "average performance levels among all people at that age who are free of known brain or other organ system diseases in terms of decline from function levels, or as adequacy to perform all activities that the individual wishes to undertake."

The brain is a complex organ and has at least three levels of functions that affect all aspects of our daily lives: interpretation of senses and control of movement; maintenance of cognitive, mental, and emotional processes; and maintenance of normal behaviour and social cognition. Brain health may therefore be defined as the preservation of optimal brain integrity and mental and cognitive function at a given age in the absence of overt brain diseases that affect normal brain function.

Effect of major neurological disorders on brain health

Several neurological disorders may disrupt brain function and affect humans' health. Medically, neurological disorders that cause brain dysfunction can be classified into three groups:

• Brain diseases with overt damage to brain structures, such as cerebrovascular diseases, traumatic brain injury, brain tumours, meningitis, and communication and sensory disorders

• Functional brain disorders with detectable destruction of brain connections or networks, such as neurodegenerative diseases (e.g., Parkinson's disease, Alzheimer's disease, and other dementias) and mental disorders (e.g., schizophrenia, depression, bipolar disorder, alcoholism, and drug abuse)

• Other brain disorders without detectable structural or functional impairment, such as migraine and sleep disorders.

These neurological disorders may have different or common effects on brain health and function. For instance, Alzheimer's disease is the main type of dementia, with a decline in different domains of cognitive function. Mood disorders may cause dysfunction in execution, reward processing, and emotional regulations. In addition to physical disability, aphasia, gait and balance problems, and cerebrovascular diseases may lead to cognitive impairment and dementia, which are neglected by both patients and physicians.

Ageing and burden of neurological disorders

Human ageing is mainly reflected in the aspects of brain ageing and degradation of brain function. The number of people aged 60 years and over worldwide was around 900 million in 2015 and is expected to grow to two billion by 2050. With the increases in population ageing and growth, the burden of neurological disorders and challenges to the preservation of brain health steeply increase. People with neurological disorders will have physical disability, cognitive or mental disorders, and social dysfunction and be a large economic burden.

Globally, neurological disorders were the leading cause of disability adjusted life years (276 million) and the second leading cause of death (9 million) in 2016, according to the Global Burden of Diseases study. Stroke, migraine, Alzheimer's disease and other dementias, and meningitis are the largest contributors to neurological disability adjusted life years. About one in four adults will have a stroke in their lifetime, from the age of 25 years onwards. Roughly 50 million people worldwide were living with dementia in 2018, and the number will more than triple to 152 million by 2050. In the following decades, governments will face increasing demand for treatment, rehabilitation, and support services for neurological disorders.

11 BEST FOODS TO BOOST YOUR BRAIN AND MEMORY

1. Fatty fish

When people talk about brain foods, fatty fish is often at the top of the list.

This type of fish includes salmon, trout, albacore tuna, herring, and sardines, all of which are rich sources of omega-3 fatty acids.

About 60% of your brain is made of fat, and half of that fat is comprised of omega-3 fatty acids.

Your brain uses omega-3s to build brain and nerve cells, and these facts are essential for learning and memory.

Omega-3s also offer several additional benefits for your brain.

For one thing, they may slow age-related mental decline and help ward off Alzheimer's disease.

On the flip side, not getting enough omega-3s is linked to learning impairments, as well as depression.

In general, eating fish seems to have positive health benefits.

Some research also suggests that people who eat fish regularly tend to have more gray matter in their brains. Gray matter contains most of the nerve cells that control decision making, memory, and emotion.

Overall, fatty fish is an excellent choice for brain health.

2. Coffee

If coffee is the highlight of your morning, you'll be glad to hear that it's good for you.

Two main components in coffee caffeine and antioxidants can help support brain health.

The caffeine found in coffee has a number of positive effects on the brain, including:

• Increased alertness. Caffeine keeps your brain alert by blocking adenosine, a chemical messenger that makes you feel sleepy.

• Improved mood. Caffeine may also boost some of your "feel-good" neurotransmitters, such as dopamine.

• Sharpened concentration. One study found that caffeine consumption led to short-term improvements in attention and alertness in participants completing a cognition test.

Drinking coffee over the long-term is also linked to a reduced risk of neurological diseases, such as Parkinson's and Alzheimer's. The largest risk reduction was seen in those adults who consumes 3-4 cups daily.

This could at least be partly due to coffee's high concentration of antioxidants.

3. Blueberries

Blueberries provide numerous health benefits, including some that are specifically for your brain.

Blueberries and other deeply colored berries deliver anthocyanins, a group of plant compounds with anti-inflammatory and antioxidant effects.

Antioxidants act against both oxidative stress and inflammation, conditions that can contribute to brain aging and neurodegenerative diseases.

Some of the antioxidants in blueberries have been found to accumulate in the brain and help improve communication between brain cells.

According to one review of 11 studies, blueberries could help improve memory and certain cognitive processes in children and older adults.

Try sprinkling them over your breakfast cereal, adding them to a smoothie, or enjoying as is for a simple snack.

4. Turmeric

Turmeric has generated a lot of buzz recently.

This deep-yellow spice is a key ingredient in curry powder and has a number of benefits for the brain.

Curcumin, the active ingredient in turmeric, has been shown to cross the blood-brain barrier, meaning it can directly enter the brain and benefit the cells there.

It's a potent antioxidant and anti-inflammatory compound that has been linked to the following brain benefits:

• May benefit memory. Curcumin may help improve memory in people with Alzheimer's. It may also help clear the amyloid plaques that are a hallmark of this disease.

• Eases depression. Curcumin boosts serotonin and dopamine, both of which improve mood. One review found that curcumin could improve symptoms of depression and anxiety when used alongside standard treatments in people diagnosed with depression.

• Helps new brain cells grow. Curcumin boosts brain-derived neurotrophic factor, a type of growth hormone that helps brain cells grow. It may help delay age-related mental decline, but more research is needed.

Keep in mind that most studies use highly concentrated curcumin supplements in doses ranging from 500–2,000 mg per day, which is much more curcumin than most people typically consume when using turmeric as a spice. This is because turmeric is only made up of around 3–6% curcumin.

Therefore, while adding turmeric to your food may be beneficial, you may need to use a curcumin supplement under a doctor's guidance to obtain the results reported in these studies.

5. Broccoli

Broccoli is packed with powerful plant compounds, including antioxidants.

It's also very high in vitamin K, delivering more than 100% of the Recommended Daily Intake (RDI) in a 1-cup (160-gram) serving of cooked broccoli.

This fat-soluble vitamin is essential for forming sphingolipids, a type of fat that's densely packed into brain cells.

A few studies in older adults have linked a higher vitamin K intake to better memory and cognitive status.

Beyond vitamin K, broccoli contains a number of compounds that give it anti-inflammatory and antioxidant effects, which may help protect the brain against damage.

6. Pumpkin seeds

Pumpkin seeds contain powerful antioxidants that protect the body and brain from free-radical damage.

They're also an excellent source of magnesium, iron, zinc, and copper.

Each of these nutrients is important for brain health:

• Zinc. This element is crucial for nerve signaling. Zinc deficiency has been linked to many neurological conditions, including Alzheimer's disease, depression, and Parkinson's disease.

• Magnesium. Magnesium is essential for learning and memory. Low magnesium levels are linked to many neurological diseases, including migraine, depression, and epilepsy.

• Copper. Your brain uses copper to help control nerve signals. And when copper levels are out of whack, there's a higher risk of neurodegenerative disorders, such as Alzheimer's.

• Iron. Iron deficiency is often characterized by brain fog and impaired brain function.

The research focuses mostly on these micronutrients, rather than pumpkin seeds themselves. However, since pumpkin seeds are high in these micronutrients, you can likely reap their benefits by adding pumpkin seeds to your diet.

7. Dark chocolate

Dark chocolate and cocoa powder are packed with a few brain-boosting compounds, including flavonoids, caffeine, and antioxidants.

Dark chocolate has a 70% or greater cocoa content. These benefits are not seen with regular milk chocolate, which contains between 10–50% cocoa.

Flavonoids are a group of antioxidant plant compounds.

The flavonoids in chocolate gather in the areas of the brain that deal with learning and memory. Researchers believe that these compounds may enhance memory and also help slow down age-related mental decline.

In fact, a number of studies back this up.

According to one study in over 900 people, those who ate chocolate more frequently performed better in a series of mental tasks, including some involving memory, compared with those who rarely ate it.

Chocolate is also a legitimate mood booster, according to research.

One study found that participants who ate chocolate experienced increased positive feelings compared to those who ate crackers.

However, it's still not clear whether that's because of compounds in the chocolate or simply because the tasty flavor makes people happy.

8. Nuts

Research has shown that eating nuts can improve heart-health markers, and having a healthy heart is linked to having a healthy brain.

One study found that regular consumption of nuts could be linked to a lower risk of cognitive decline in older adults.

Also, another 2014 study found that women who ate nuts regularly over the course of several years had a sharper memory compared with those who did not eat nuts.

Several nutrients in nuts, such as healthy fats, antioxidants, and vitamin E, may explain their beneficial effects on brain health.

Vitamin E protects cells against free-radical damage to help slow mental decline.

While all nuts are good for your brain, walnuts may have an extra edge, since they also deliver anti-inflammatory omega-3 fatty acids.

9. Oranges

You can get almost all the vitamin C you need in a day by eating one medium orange.

Doing so is important for brain health since vitamin C is a key factor in preventing mental decline.

According to one study, having higher levels of vitamin C in the blood was associated with improvements in tasks involving focus, memory, attention, and decision speed.

Vitamin C is a powerful antioxidant that helps fight off the free radicals that can damage brain cells. Plus, vitamin C supports brain health as you age and may protect against conditions like major depressive disorder, anxiety, schizophrenia, and Alzheimer's disease.

You can also get high amounts of vitamin C from other foods like bell peppers, guava, kiwi, tomatoes, and strawberries.

10. Eggs

Eggs are a good source of several nutrients tied to brain health, including vitamins B6 and B12, folate, and choline.

Choline is an important micronutrient that your body uses to create acetylcholine, a neurotransmitter that helps regulate mood and memory.

Two older studies found that higher intakes of choline were linked to better memory and mental function.

Nevertheless, many people do not get enough choline in their diet.

Eating eggs is an easy way to get choline, given that egg yolks are among the most concentrated sources of this nutrient.

Adequate intake of choline is 425 mg per day for most women and 550 mg per day for men, with just a single egg yolk containing 112 mg.

Furthermore, the B vitamins found in eggs also have several roles in brain health.

To start, they may help slow the progression of mental decline in older adults by lowering levels of homocysteine, an amino acid that could be linked to dementia and Alzheimer's disease.

Also, being deficient in two types of B vitamins folate and B12 has been linked to depression.

Folate deficiency is common in older people with dementia, and studies show that folic acid supplements can help minimize age-related mental decline.

Vitamin B12 is also involved in synthesizing brain chemicals and regulating sugar levels in the brain.

It's worth noting that there's very little direct research on the link between eating eggs and brain health. However, there is research to support the brain-boosting benefits of the specific nutrients found in eggs.

11. Green tea

As is the case with coffee, the caffeine in green tea boosts brain function.

In fact, it has been found to improve alertness, performance, memory, and focus.

But green tea also has other components that make it a brain-healthy beverage.

One of them is L-theanine, an amino acid that can cross the blood-brain barrier and increase the activity of the neurotransmitter GABA, which helps reduce anxiety and makes you feel more relaxed.

L-theanine also increases the frequency of alpha waves in the brain, which helps you relax without making you feel tired.

One review found that the L-theanine in green tea can help you relax by counteracting the stimulating effects of caffeine.

It's also rich in polyphenols and antioxidants that could protect the brain from mental decline and reduce the risk of Alzheimer's and Parkinson's.

Plus, some studies have shown green tea helps improve memory.

CHAPTER THREE

BRAIN HEALTH RECIPES

Almost all the food we eat is good for the brain because the brain controls everything in the body, so here are some of so many recipes you can eat to boost brain ability, and each of the recipes are explained in details by listing the ingredients alongside the instructions on how to go about it;

Orange Cream

Ingredients

20-24 Medjool dates

vegan dark chocolate , Enjoy Life Dark Chocolate Chips

For the Cashew Cream:

1 cup raw unsalted cashews , soaked in water for ~2-3 hours then drain and discard the water)

1 cup shredded unsweetened coconut

1/2 cup orange juice , freshly squeezed if possible

1/2 teasp vanilla extract

pure maple syrup , optional

For Garnish:

orange zest

shredded coconut

sea salt

Instructions

To Make the Orange Cream:

Add the soaked and drained cashews, unsweetened shredded coconut, orange juice, and vanilla extract into a blender (such as a Vitamix).

Blend completely until thick, creamy, and slightly chunky (I used my tamper for this process). This should not take too long. Stop once you feel like all of the cashews are completely blended in. Do not blend too long otherwise you will start to make cashew butter.

Depending on the sweetness of the orange juice and your preference, you may or may-not need a little maple syrup blended into the cream for some added sweetness. Note that this cream should not be overly sweet since it's being stuffed into dates (see notes below). Set the orange cream aside.

To Prepare the Dates:

You have one of two options: (1) Cut a thin section across the wide end of the date to cut the end. Using clean sharp tweezers, going in from the cut end, pull out the pit to create a port to stuff. OR (2) Using a knife, make an incision across the length of the date and carefully remove the pit, creating a 'boat' to stuff. (see notes below)

To Stuff the Dates:

If using option (1) above, using a condiment dispenser , piping bag , or syringe, completely fill the hole created inside the date with the prepared orange cream. If using option (2) above, use a small spoon or knife to stuff the dates where you made the incision. With this option, you will stuff more of the orange cream and it will be visible on top. (see pictures above)

Once you've stuffed the dates with orange cream, melt the dark chocolate chips over a double broiler or in small increments in the microwave.

Line a baking sheet or plate with wax paper. If using option (1) above, simply dip the dates half way up covering the open side of the date. If using option (2) above, simply drizzle the melted chocolate across the dates on top of the stuffed orange cream.

Place on the prepared plate/baking sheet, sprinkle the top of the dates with a tiny amount of orange zest, unsweetened shredded coconut, and/or sea salt, and place in the fridge until the chocolate is completely solidified.

Store in the fridge in an airtight container until ready to enjoy!

Green Banana Flour Brownie Bites

You'd never guess that these luscious, super chocolaty, brownie bites are made with belly friendly green banana flour which helps promote a healthy, happy gut microbiome, along with other resistant starch foods.

Ingredients

1/4 cup vegan dark chocolate chips

1/2 cup green banana flour , i.e. Let's Do Organic Green Banana Flour

1/2 cup chopped pecans

1/4 cup unsweetened cocoa

2 tablespoons pure maple syrup, or to taste

2-3+ tablespoons almond milk, or other non-dairy milk

1 teaspoon pure vanilla extract

1/4 teaspoon salt

Instructions

Melt chocolate chips in the a small microwave safe bowl, on high power, in the microwave for 1 minute. Stir, and microwave for an additional 30 seconds, or until chocolate chips are fully melted. Set aside and allow to cool slightly.

Combine banana flour, chopped pecans, cocoa, maple syrup, almond milk, vanilla extract, and salt in the bowl of a food processor. Process for 1 minutes then add melted chocolate chips to mixture, and process for an additional 2-3 minutes, stopping to scrape side of bowl as needed, until mixture is very fine fine and crumbly.

Using clean hands, form mixture into 8 ~ 1 inch balls, and place them on a serving dish, or in a storage container. If not consuming all of the Brownie Bites right away, you can store them in the refrigerator in a sealed container for up to 3 days, or in the freezer for up to 1 week,

Soft Amaretti Cookies

There are infinite variations of this classic Italian cookie. I'd like to share this simple, gluten free recipe for Soft Amaretti Cookies with all of you.

Ingredients

250 grams almond flour scant 2 1/2 cups

200 grams sugar approx 1 cup

lemon zest of one medium lemon

3 egg whites

1 teaspoon bitter almond extract

extra granulated sugar for rolling sprinkle 1/3 cup in a large dinner plate, set aside

Instructions

Preheat oven to 325° F. Position rack in the center.

Line large baking sheet with parchment paper.

In a large bowl, whisk almond flour and sugar together.

Add grated lemon zest and whisk a few more times. Set aside.

In a separate bowl, whisk egg whites to a soft peak stage.

Whisk in the bitter almond extract.

Gently incorporate the egg whites to the dry ingredients. Once the dough is completely moist, you are done.

Use the smallest ice cream scooper to portion the dough (about 1 tablespoon).

With slightly damp hands, press your palms into the plate of sugar.

Roll each ball of dough with your sugar coated palms and then again in the sugar found on the plate.

Place on the paper lined baking sheet.

Bake for about 25 minutes or until bottoms are golden brown in color.

Cool before storing at room temperature in airtight containers. Will keep for 3-4 days.

Moroccan Lentils With Turkey Meatballs

Ingredients

FOR THE TURKEY MEATBALLS:

1 pound ground turkey

1 egg

½ cup bread crumbs

3 tablespoons parsley, chopped

3 garlic cloves, minced

1 teaspoon cumin

1 teaspoon paprika

½ teaspoon turmeric

¼ teaspoon ground cloves

¼ teaspoon cayenne

½ teaspoon salt

½ teaspoon pepper

FOR THE LENTILS:

2 tablespoons olive oil

3 garlic cloves, minced

1 medium yellow onion, diced

3 medium carrots, thinly sliced

1 teaspoon cumin

1 teaspoon paprika

½ teaspoon turmeric

¼ teaspoon cayenne, (optional)

¼ teaspoon ground cloves

½ teaspoon salt

½ teaspoon pepper

1 cup green or brown lentils

4 cups chicken stock

14.5 ounces petite diced tomatoes (canned)

3 tablespoons parsley chopped,, plus more for garnish

Instructions

Preheat oven to 350F.

Combine the turkey, egg, bread crumbs, fresh parsley, minced garlic, and meatball spices in a large bowl. Mix together without overworking.

Form fifteen 2-inch meatballs and place them on a parchment-lined baking sheet. Bake in a preheated 350 degree oven for 10 minutes.

Meanwhile, start the lentils: in a large pan saute the garlic, onion and carrots in olive oil for 8-10 minutes over medium heat. Stir in the lentil spices, then add lentils and chicken stock. Bring to a simmer and cook for 18-20 minutes uncovered.

Add in diced tomatoes, parsley, and baked meatballs, and continue to simmer for 10 more minutes.

Garnish with more chopped parsley and serve.

Ginger Turmeric Chicken

Ingredients

2 inch piece fresh ginger, peeled

1 inch piece fresh turmeric, peeled or 1 teaspoon powder turmeric

4 cloves garlic

1 tablespoon cumin

1 tablespoon paprika

1 teaspoon dried oregano

3 tablespoons olive oil

3 tablespoons apple cider vinegar

2 tablespoons coconut aminos, (low sodium tamari or soy sauce can also be used)

2 lbs boneless skinless chicken thighs*

sea salt, to taste

sweet red peppers, for garnish (optional)

Instructions

Prepare Marinade

Combine ginger, turmeric, garlic, cumin, paprika, dried oregano, olive oil, apple cider vinegar and coconut aminos in a food processor or blender. Process to make a thick paste

Add marinade to 2 lbs chicken thighs in a glass bowl (or ziplock bag) and marinade overnight in refrigerator

Grill Ginger Turmeric Chicken

Heat gas grill to medium heat

Remove chicken from marinade and place on the grill turning occasionally until fully cooked, about 12-14 minutes depending on the heat of your grill

Sprinkle lightly with sea salt and serve

Quinoa Tabbouleh

You can whip up a batch of this fresh and easy quinoa tabbouleh {gluten free, low FODMAP, vegan} in 20 minutes! Enjoy it for dinner with your favorite sides, then save the leftovers for lunch the next day. It's nourishing AND delicious!

Ingredients

1 cup dry quinoa, rinsed if needed

2 cups water

2 large cucumbers, peeled and chopped into bite size pieces

2 cups grape or cherry tomatoes, sliced into bite size pieces

2 cups loosely packed flat leaf parsley, chopped

1 cup chopped green onions, green part only

1 cup loosely packed fresh mint, chopped

1/4 cup lemon juice

1/4 cup extra virgin olive oil

1 teaspoon dried oregano

Salt and Pepper to taste

Instructions

Rinse the quinoa if not pre-rinsed. Place in a medium pot with water, and heat on high until boiling. Turn the heat down to a simmer, and cook for ~ 15 minutes.

While the quinoa is cooking, peel and chop the cucumbers and slice the tomatoes. Place them in a large salad bowl or serving dish. Add the chopped parsley, green onions, and mint to the cucumber and tomatoes, and stir well to combine.

Juice the lemon and add to the herbs and veggies along with the olive oil.

When quinoa has finished cooking, pour it into the bowl with the other ingredients, and stir well to combine. Stir in the dried oregano, and salt and pepper to taste.

Serve warm, or chilled {store covered in refrigerator until ready to serve, or for up to 3 days.

Lentil Salad With Lemon Vinaigrette

Ingredients

2 cups chopped kale

3/4 cup cherry tomatoes, sliced in half

1/2 cup chopped Radicchio

1/2 cup cooked lentils

2 tablespoons slivered almonds

1 tablespoon extra virgin olive oil

Juice from 1/4 of a lemon

Sea salt and black pepper to taste

Instructions

Place kale, cherry tomatoes, optional Radicchio, lentils, and almonds in a salad bowl. Top with olive oil, lemon juice, and salt and pepper to taste. Toss well, then serve.

Asian Pan Seared Salmon Salad for One

Ingredients

1 6- ounce wild salmon filet

1 cup chopped Napa cabbage

1/4 cup chopped green onion

1/8 cup peanuts

1 teaspoon Golden Balsamic vinegar

2 teaspoons extra virgin olive oil, divided

1 teaspoons sesame oil

1 teaspoon Braggs Amino Acids or gluten-free Tamari

1/4 teaspoon Chinese 5 Spice Powder, or to taste

salt and pepper

Instructions

Heat a large heavy skillet over medium heat, add peanuts, and cook for ~3 minutes, stirring constantly to prevent burning. Remove peanuts from skillet, and allow to cool.

Add 1 teaspoon oil to the same skillet, and place salmon filet, skin side down, in the pan. Sprinkle salt and pepper on top and cook for 4 minutes, then flip over and cook for another 3 minutes. Remove salmon from pan to cool.

While salmon is cooking, chop the Napa cabbage and onions up, and make the dressing by combining the remaining olive oil with the sesame oil, balsamic vinegar, Braggs Amino Acids, and the Chinese 5 Spice Powder. Stir well, and set aside.

Assemble the salad by placing the cabbage on a plate, top with the salmon filet, sprinkle the green onions and peanuts on top, then drizzle the dressing over the salad.

Greek Yogurt Parfait, Bananas Foster Style

This easy, healthy Greek Yogurt Parfait is made with a delicious twist! Greek yogurt is paired with scrumptious bananas foster and a nourishing cinnamon flax nut streusel topping. Make it for a protein & fiber packed breakfast or afternoon snack!

Ingredients

1/4 cup pecans or walnuts, or any nuts of choice

2 tablespoons ground flaxseed meal

1/2 teaspoon cinnamon, divided

2 teaspoons vegan spread, i.e. Earth Balance

2 bananas, peeled and sliced in to 1/4 inch rounds

2 teaspoons maple syrup

1 1/3 cup plain Greek yogurt

Instructions

For Streusel: Combine walnuts, flax meal, 2 teaspoons brown sugar, and 1/4 teaspoon cinnamon in food processor. Pulse ingredients together until walnuts are very finely chopped. Set aside. {Note: You can make a large batch of this ahead of time and store it in the fridge.}

For Bananas: Heat coconut oil in sauté pan then add sliced bananas and cook on medium heat for approximately 1 minute. Sprinkle bananas with remaining cinnamon and brown sugar, then reduce heat to low and cook for approximately one more minute, or until bananas are nice and caramelized.

For each serving, place 1/2 cup Greek yogurt in a cup or bowl, then top with bananas and cinnamon streusel mixture.

Enjoy!

Blueberry Smoothie Bowl

Ingredients

1/3 cup Seven Sundays Blueberry Chia Buckwheat Muesli

1/2 cup organic soymilk, unsweetened; add extra if needed

1 cup blueberries, fresh or frozen

1 tablespoon ground flaxseed

1/4 teaspoon ground ginger

pinch of salt

1 kiwi fruit, peeled and sliced

1 tablespoon hemp seeds

viola flowers, optional

Instructions

Combine all ingredients EXCEPT the hemp seeds, kiwi fruit, and viola flowers, in a blender. Blend on high speed to combine well. Add additional milk if needed, to thin the consistency.

Pour smoothie into a serving bowl. Top with sliced kiwi fruit, hemp seeds, and viola flowers.

Falafel Waffle

Ingredients

Waffle

1 (15 oz.) can chickpeas (also know as garbanzo beans), rinsed and drained

1 small bunch scallions, sliced

1 Tbsp. parsley, chopped

2 Tbsp. cilantro, chopped

3 cloves garlic, minced

1 tsp. cumin

½ tsp. coriander

¼ tsp. cayenne pepper (use 1/8 tsp. if you don't like spicy)

1 tsp. baking powder

3 eggs, lightly beaten

3 Tbsp. garbanzo flour (all-purpose flour works too, if you are not gluten free)

Salt & freshly ground pepper, to taste

Sauce

¾ cup plain Greek yogurt

1-2 Tbsp. tahini

1 tsp. chili garlic sauce

½ lemon, zest & juice

Garnish

½ diced tomato

¼ cup diced cucumber

Lemon wedge

Instructions

Preheat waffle iron. (High setting if you waffle maker has this option.)

In a food processor bowl, add the chickpeas, scallions, parsley, cilantro, garlic, cumin, coriander, cayenne, and baking powder. Pulse to combine until finely chopped. Season with salt and pepper to taste.

Add the eggs and pulse to combine. Add the flour until combined.

Grease the waffle iron with cooking spray. Add batter to waffle iron and cook 4-5 minutes until golden-brown and crispy. (Cook until there is no steam, don't peak too early or the waffle will separate.)

For the yogurt sauce:

In a small bowl add all sauce ingredients, mix well. If you like your mixture thinner, just add a little water.

Garnish:

Sprinkle with diced tomato & cucumber, and lemon wedge on the side. (Alternative, mix the tomato & cucumber into the yogurt sauce.)

Cantaloup Breakfast Bowl

Ingredients

1 whole cantaloupe

1 1/2 cups cottage cheese

1 cup blueberries

1/4 cup pecans, chopped

2 tbsp hemp seeds

Instructions

Wash cantaloupe and pat dry. Slice in half and scoop out seeds.

Fill each cantaloupe half with 3/4 cup cottage cheese, then top each hald off with 1/2 cup blueberries, 2 tablespoons chopped pecans, and 1 tablespoon hemp seeds. Enjoy!

Red Pepper, Kale And Feta Frittata

Ingredients

Oil spray

3 cloves garlic, minced

1 medium red bell pepper, diced

2 cups kale, chopped

½ cup feta cheese crumbles

8 large eggs

½ cup skim milk

¼ teaspoon freshly cracked black pepper

¼ teaspoon sea salt

Instructions

Heat oven to 350°F. Generously spray a pie dish with oil.

Spread garlic, red peppers and kale in the pie dish. Sprinkle feta over vegetables.

In a medium bowl, whisk eggs, milk, pepper and salt. Pour mixture over kale and feta in the pie dish.

Bake 25 to 35 minutes, or until eggs are set. Remove from oven and serve, or cool before storing in the refrigerator, covered.

Mediterranean Omelette

A quick, easy and satisfying omelette they is brimming with tasty Mediterranean inspired flavours!

ingredients

1 teaspoon oil or butter

2 eggs

1 tablespoon milk (or cream)

oregano, salt and pepper to taste

2 tablespoons tomato, diced

2 tablespoons kalamata olives, sliced

1 artichoke heart, quartered

1 tablespoon feta, crumbled

1 tablespoon romesco sauce

directions

Heat the oil in a small skillet (no-stick preferable), pour in the mixture of the egg, milk, oregano, salt and pepper and let cover the bottom of the pan.

Cook until the egg starts to set before sprinkling on the tomato, olive, artichoke and feta per half of the egg and folding the covered part over.

Cook the eggs until set, about a minute, before removing from the heat and topping with the romesco sauce to enjoy!

Baked Shakshuka With Fennel And Goat Cheese

Ingredients

1 tablespoon extra virgin olive oil

1/2 medium onion diced

1 bulb fennel chopped

2 cloves garlic crushed

1 teaspoon smoked paprika ground

1 1/2 teaspoons cumin ground

1 28 ounce can diced tomatoes no salt added preferred

6 large eggs

2 ounces goat cheese crumbled or sliced

1 tablespoon fresh rosemary chopped

Instructions

Preheat oven to 400 degrees Farenheit.

In a 10" (or larger) cast iron skillet, heat olive oil on medium heat. Saute the onions and and fennel cook until softening, about 5-7 minutes.

Stir in garlic and spices and cook for an additional minute to make aromatic.

Add the tomatoes and bring to a simmer. Cook until the liquid thickens, up to 10 minutes. Crack the eggs over the pan and distribute evenly over the pan (can do 5 eggs around the edge and 1 egg in the middle).

Sprinkle the goat cheese and rosemary on top. Slowly transfer the dish to the oven. Bake for up to 10 minutes or until the middle of the eggs are set. Check at the 5 minute mark if you prefer runny eggs. For harder, cooked eggs cook a little longer than 10 minutes.

Top with additional fresh rosemary or other herbs.

Lemon Basil Chickpea Fritters

Ingredients

15-ounce can chickpeas, drained and rinsed

2 tablespoons (20 milliliters) lemon juice

¼ cup whole-wheat flour

½ teaspoon salt

¼ cup shredded Parmesan cheese

3 tablespoons fresh basil, chopped

1 teaspoon lemon zest

1 tablespoon (14 milliliters) avocado oil

Instructions

In a large bowl, stir together chickpeas, lemon juice, flour and salt. Mash with potato masher or fork until a thick paste is formed, leaving a few chickpeas whole for texture. Stir in Parmesan cheese, basil and lemon zest.

With clean hands, form mixture into 6 golf ball-sized balls. Flatten into patties, roughly 2 inches to 3 inches in diameter. Place on a plate.

In a large skillet, heat oil over medium-high heat. Add 3 to 4 patties to skillet, being mindful not to overcrowd the pan.

Cook one side for 1 to 2 minutes, or until golden brown and crispy. Flip and cook for an additional 1 to 2 minutes. Transfer to a towel-lined plate.

Cook remaining patties and serve immediately.

Stuffed Acorn Squash With Spiced Rice

Ingredients

Acorn Squash

2 acorn squash

2 tablespoons olive oil

1/2 teaspoon allspice

1/2 teaspoon Kosher salt

Rice Stuffing

2 tablespoon ghee divided

1/2-pound ground beef

1/2 small red onion chopped finely

1 garlic clove chopped finely

1/2 teaspoon cinnamon

1/2 teaspoon cumin

1/4 teaspoon allspice

Pinch of nutmeg

1/4 teaspoon Kosher salt

Black pepper

1/2 cup uncooked Basmati rice washed and rinsed

3/4 cup low sodium chicken stock

1/4 cup pine nuts

1/3 cup dried cranberries (or dried currants

Fresh parsley leaves roughly chopped

Instructions

Pre-heat Oven: Start by preheating the oven to 400 degrees Fahrenheit and wash and dry the acorn squash.

Prep Acorn Squash: Cut squash in half, horizontally and scoop out any seeds. You may need to cut a small piece of the bottom off so the squash can stand up without topping over.

Roast Squash: Brush olive oil all over the inside of the flesh and season with allspice and salt. Place squash on a foil lined backing sheet cut side down and roast for 25-30 minutes until just barely cooked through. Once done, remove from the oven and let cool slightly.

Make Rice Filling: While the squash roasts, make the spiced rice filling. Heat a pot over medium heat and melt 1 tablespoon of ghee. Add ground beef and onion and cook until meat is filly cooked through and onion has softened.

Add garlic and spices and give everything a good saute.

Add basmati rice and give everything another stir and pour in stock. Add 1 tablespoon of ghee and bring to a boil then reduce to a simmer. Cook until rice is cooked through, about 15 minutes.

Toast the Pine Nuts: While rice cooks, make the toasted pine nuts. Melt ghee in a small skillet and add pine nuts. Saute until pine nuts just begin to toast and turn golden brown and small nutty. Remove from heat and set aside, they will be very hot.

Once rice is done, fluff with a fork and add toasted pine nuts, dried cranberries and chopped parsley.

Stuff Squash with Filling: Add a heaping half cup of filling to squash, depending how large your squash are and lightly drizzle the tops with olive oil.

Finish Cooking Squash: Place back in the oven and continue roasting until squash is fully cooked, another 20 minutes. You may need to cover with foil so the tops don't get too dark too quickly.

Once done, let cool slightly before serving and garnish with extra fresh herbs.

Mediterranean Kale Salad

Ingredients

1 tomato, diced

2 thinly sliced roasted red peppers

6 cups lightly packed, de-stemmed and finely chopped kale

1 medium zucchini, diced

1 cucumber, diced

1 19 oz. can chickpeas, drained and well-rinsed

3/4 cup pitted kalmata olives (about 40 olives or 10 per serving)

1 small white onion, diced

3 cloves garlic, minced

3 tbsp balsamic vinegar

2 tbsp fresh lemon juice

1 tbsp pure maple syrup

1 tbsp extra virgin olive oil

1 tsp dried rosemary

2 tsp dried oregano

2 tsp dried basil

1 tsp garlic powder

1 tsp sea salt

1 tsp black pepper

optional: tofu feta

Instructions

Place everything into a large bowl and mix well.

Serve right away. Leftovers can be stored in the fridge up to 3 days.

Mediterranean Turkey Stuffed Eggplant

Ingredients

2 medium eggplants

Olive oil

1 cup chopped onion (from 1 small onion)

3 garlic cloves, minced

1 lb. ground turkey

1 ½ tsp oregano

1 tsp paprika

½ tsp salt

¼ tsp pepper

¼ tsp cinnamon

¾ cup chopped tomatoes (from 1 small tomato), plus more for topping

⅓ cup halved kalamata olives

⅓ cup crumbled feta cheese

¾ cup Hood Sour Cream, plus more for topping

¼ cup panko

¼ cup chopped parsley, for garnish

Instructions

Pre-heat oven to 350 degrees.

Slice eggplants in half lengthwise. Leaving about a ½ inch border around the edges and cutting deep but taking care not to pierce skin, score eggplant flesh diagonally one way and then diagonally the other way to form a diamond pattern. Brush each eggplant half with 1 tsp olive oil, ⅛ tsp salt, and ⅛ tsp pepper.

Place eggplant halves on baking sheet and bake for about 30 minutes, until flesh is golden. Remove from oven to let cool a bit.

When eggplants are cool enough to touch scoop out the flesh and chop it into cubes.

Heat 1 Tbsp olive oil in a large skillet over medium heat. Add onion and cook for 4-5 minutes until translucent. Add garlic and cook for 2 more minutes.

Add turkey to skillet, along with oregano, paprika, salt, pepper, and cinnamon. Cook turkey, breaking up with a spatula or fork, until cooked through. Drain excess oil from skillet if necessary. Stir in tomatoes, olives, feta, and chopped eggplant and cook for another minute.

Remove skillet from heat and stir in Hood Sour Cream.

Stuff eggplants with turkey mixture and sprinkle panko over the top of each eggplant.

Bake at 350 for about 15 minutes. Then turn broiler on and broil for 2-3 minutes, until tops of eggplants are golden.

Garnish eggplants with chopped parsley, additional chopped tomato, and additional sour cream if desired.

SUMMARY

Don't forget that as well as a healthy diet, exercise helps to keep our brains sharp. Research suggests that regular exercise improves cognitive function, slows down the mental aging process and helps us process information more effectively.

While moderate alcohol intake can have some positive health effects, excessive consumption can lead to memory loss, behavioral changes and sleep disruption. Particularly high-risk groups include teenagers, young adults and pregnant women. Processed foods contribute to excess fat around the organs, which is associated with a decline in brain tissue. Additionally, Western-style diets may increase brain inflammation and impair memory, learning, brain plasticity and the blood-brain barrier.

If your diet is unbalanced for whatever reason, you may want to consider a multivitamin and mineral complex and an omega-3 fatty acid supplement to help make up a few of the essentials. If you are considering taking a supplement it is best to discuss this with your GP or qualified healthcare professional.

The bottom line

Many foods can help keep your brain healthy.

Some foods, such as the fruits and vegetables in this list, as well as tea and coffee, have antioxidants that help protect your brain from damage.

Others, such as nuts and eggs, contain nutrients that support memory and brain development.

You can help support your brain health and boost your alertness, memory, and mood by strategically including these foods in your diet.

Just one thing. Try this today: Just as important as including these brain-boosting foods in your diet is steering clear of foods that can negatively impact brain health.

www.ingramcontent.com/pod-product-compliance
Lightning Source LLC
Chambersburg PA
CBHW050048260726
48658CB00005B/1835